Heal your skin

easily, quickly, affordably and naturally.

Marie D.M.

To my wonderful friend Erica C., with love.

Disclaimer

THIS BOOK DOES NOT PROVIDE MEDICAL ADVICE

The information, including but not limited to, text, graphics, images and other material contained in this book are for informational purposes only. The purpose of this book is to promote broad consumer understanding and knowledge of various health topics. It is not intended to be a substitute for professional medical advice, diagnosis or treatment. Always seek the advice of your physician or other qualified health care provider with any questions you may have regarding a medical condition or treatment and before undertaking a new health care regimen, and never disregard professional medical advice or delay in seeking it because of something you have read on this book.

Table Of Contents

Introduction: my acne story

A couple of weeks ago, I was riding the metro into the city on a Saturday night when I saw a young blonde girl come in. She was beautiful and in great shape, but had severe, angry cystic acne, just like mine once was. Unlike me, she hadn't caked on makeup to conceal it. I watched as she looked at herself in the train's window, and tried to telepathically communicate to her the method I used to heal my acne (if you're wondering why I didn't strike up a conversation with her, well… when I had acne, I was feeling too vulnerable to take the unsolicited advice of strangers well! I didn't want to risk making her feel as terrible as I once felt).

That brief encounter made me think of my own acne story, and on how I wish I knew there was an easier, faster, less expensive and natural way to make it go away.

From the moment I hit puberty, acne immediately showed its ugly head. During my teens, I was determined to hide any evidence of pimples I failed to obliterate with the multiple-step treatments I spent all my babysitting money on. I wouldn't leave the house until my face was caked with makeup and my hair pin-straight (accumulating a record number of late slips that, today, I'm half-proud, half-ashamed of).

If I obsessed over the blemishes I had in high school, I had no idea what was still in store for me. A few months before I left for college, I felt a painful bump on my cheek, right under my eye. For weeks, there was nothing I could do about it. My attempt to pop it only made it bigger, redder in colour, and more difficult to hide with makeup.

When I started college appeared on my forehead, and then a couple more on my cheeks. I was referred by the college health counsellor to a doctor who put me on the birth control pill, promising it would solve my acne problem in no time. Instead, it made it worse. In the space of two weeks, my face was covered with painful, pus-filled blisters, along with groups of whiteheads and patches of dry, angry skin. All the makeup in the world couldn't completely hide that. And as you can imagine, being essentially disfigured a terrible toll on me. I went from a confident, hot young girl to one who was being ghosted after first dates, getting turned away by nightclub bouncers, and pointed at by children in public transportation. That made me sink into depression, and by the end of my first year of college, I felt so defeated that I decided to take a leave of absence to focus on healing my acne.

I returned home and immediately booked an appointment with Doctor O., a dermatologist who was reputed to be the best in my area. After I was made to wait for ages in an exam room, the doctor came in, took a quick look at my face, and said, or rather grunted at me, "I'm putting you on Acutane." I tried to understand a little bit more, as I'd only heard scary things about that treatment, but all the doctor said was that he couldn't tell me whether it would work or not.

Doctor O. left the the exam room after having seen me for about two minutes and a half, and a nurse proceeded to explain to me that I needed to decide a contraception method before I could get my prescription, because Acutane could cause severe birth defects should I get pregnant. Having landed into this mess because of a pill and not exactly having sexual partners lining up, I found myself signing an abstinence pledge. I nonetheless had to consent to monthly blood tests, because, to add insult to injury, my word that I hadn't had unprotected sex during my treatment wasn't enough.

Several months into the treatment, I didn't see any improvement. Doctor O. was still as unsympathetic (his biography on the clinic's website said he had been a surgeon in the U.S. Navy for most of his life, but it wasn't an excuse to have so little manners, especially around vulnerable patients!). All I got from Acutane were the side effects: dryness everywhere, nosebleeds, more acne acne, insomnia, and a worsening depression that made me feel increasingly hopeless I'd ever retrieve the beautiful, flawless skin I had as a child.

One evening, as I finished the cup of lavender camomile herbal tea I had made myself, a childhood memory came back to me of my grandmother swiping used tea bags on her eyes and face. I thought, *what do I have to lose?* and I did the very same with my tea bag before tossing it.

The next morning, when I walked to my vanity table to spackle on my daily dose of makeup (I then used products made for burn victims!), I immediately noticed something different. My pimples were still there, but it seemed like they were less swollen. My skin was less red than usual, my complexion more even than it had been in years.

I went to my monthly appointment with Doctor O. that afternoon, and the surprise was visible on his usually impassible, stony face. He cracked a rare smile as he said that he wasn't expecting to see such improvement. I mentioned the lavender tea, and he shrugged, saying, "those things can help too."

(I would find out, after asking a different dermatologist a few years later, that Doctor O. had prescribed me a dose that was, given my height and body weight, too low to be really effective. So all of these months of hopelessness and depression, of sickening side-effects, of dehumanising and slut-shaming pregnancy tests had been essentially for nothing.)

After I left his clinic that day, I drove to Whole Foods and bought myself a bottle of lavender essential oil. That was the turning point in my acne story.

Two weeks later, on my twentieth birthday, I was able to not wear make-up for the first time since I hit puberty. Okay, I did wear some mascara and lipstick; it was a festive occasion after all. But I didn't need to cake on the green primer, concealer, high-coverage cream foundation and setting powder like every day for the past two years or so. I felt a deep sense of pure joy and freedom I thought I'd never feel again.

Of course, my skin didn't remain entirely clear at first. The cysts were still there despite having retreated under my skin, and they would sometimes reappear or become more painful. I also dealt with hormonal acne, which would worsen the week before my period, and then take two more weeks to heal before coming back all over again.

But I knew that it was only a matter of time, and I could see the improvement. My first round of Acutane came to its end, and I didn't return to Doctor O.'s for another one (I had to wait a few months to prevent liver damage and other problems). Throughout the next few months, I took it upon myself to heal my skin naturally, and believing it was possible, I tested many more methods and natural products until I found what worked best for me.

It took me two years of ups and down for my skin to become almost 99.99% clear, which it has remained until this day. During that time, I also made lifestyle changes that I think were as important in my skin's healing as the products I used.

What I can guarantee you is that the method I'll talk about in the next few chapters will be **easy, affordable, quick and natural**.

It will be **easy** because there will be no need for doctor appointments, prescriptions (including those that require blood tests and abstinence pledges) and overall hassle.

It will be **affordable** because the ingredients we are re using are accessible and much less expensive than multiple-step regimens, doctor's visits, prescription medication that will cost you thousands and won't always be covered by insurance.

It will be **quick** because you will likely see and feel positive results faster than with a conventional cure, that typically will make your skin worse before it get better.

And it will be **natural** because we'll be using only organic ingredients, as opposed to harsh synthetic chemicals that mess up your hormones and come with terrible side-effects.

So let's get to it, then!

Chapter One

Acne myths, problems of conventional treatments, and how to make an informed decision.

Let me start this chapter by saying that no matter what some people might say to you, your acne is not your fault. You did not bring this upon yourself by wearing makeup, and dyeing your hair in your teens, eating chocolate, drinking too much coffee, or anything else. Acne happens to everyone, it's part of how our bodies are engineered. What we can control is what we do with this acne to make it go away. Because it does go away, faster for some of us than others, but it does heal eventually.

The biggest acne myth out there (and the reason why people suffer from acne longer than they should) is that oil causes acne. If you look at cures for acne from past decades or centuries, you'll realise that the main ingredient in DIY remedies is more than often an oil or fat. We may remember the jars of Ponds Cold Cream (an emulsion of mineral oil) our grandmothers used to cleanse their faces; in fact my eighty-year-old grandmother credits that miraculous product for making her look like she's still in her sixties.

While acne occurs when hair follicles become clogged with sebum (an oily substance produced by the skin), using oil and oil-based products to cleanse and treat your skin will not cause your acne. Your skin produces excess sebum is when it is under attack. When you use products that dry your skin out, it becomes more irritated, and your acne worsens. When you use a natural oil to nurture your skin, it takes the hydration and nourishment it needs, and the irritation calms down.

That brings us to the conventional treatments that are pushed towards teenagers and adults suffering from acne. I have tried everything, from over-the-counter treatments to prescription medication, and here's what happened. Over-the-counter treatments caused my skin to become dry, itchy, burning and peeling. All antibiotic creams and gels did (aside from more peeling and burning) was to lead to antibiotic resistance. As to oral medication, it did improve my skin a bit, but the side-effects were terrible.

Sometimes, I find myself wondering if the skincare industry pushes (among others, by means of aggressive advertising) treatments that don't work because it makes more money if people still suffer from acne. But I'm not really a conspiracy theorist, so I'll just recommend you view conventional treatments with skepticism and use common sense when making any decision regarding your health.

One thing I do not recommend doing is discontinuing your conventional treatment without talking to your doctor first. Suddenly stopping any kind of medication can be dangerous. I hope you have a doctor who takes the time to answer your questions, who takes your side-effects seriously, and who is open to natural alternatives. Consider you following both conventional and natural treatments side-by-side; it is, in fact, what I did until I finished my nine-month round of Acutane. Also, research, research, and research some more. Reach out to people who suffered from acne, whether in person or online, and ask them questions.

Test out different treatments to see what works for you. Ask older relatives or friends what worked for them; you'd be surprised at how much different old remedies were. Research everything, including all the ingredients you're planning to use. Natural ingredients can be as potent, if not more, as medication that comes out of a lab. If you're taking medication or undergoing treatment for a different condition, consult with your doctor before using any kind of essential oils; some essential oils can interfere with your medication. Same if you are pregnant or breastfeeding. Before applying any kind of product to your skin, especially undiluted essential oils, make sure to do a skin patch test to rule out the possibility for intolerance or allergies.

A word on makeup: **it doesn't cause acne.** As long as you remove it at the end of the day and properly cleanse and treat your skin, makeup will not affect your acne. Don't feel guilty for wearing some; in fact, if you suffer from acne, I say, let makeup be your greatest ally. Allow it to be your way to regain control over your condition. Turn makeup into a mindful ritual that allows you to indulge in femininity, making it an art. Let it help you feel confident, beautiful, and sexy. And talented too, because when you spend your evenings watching countless YouTube tutorials to hide severe acne and use illusion tricks to make your best features stand out, you gain skills that could rival with top makeup artists. (Check out **this video** by the gorgeous model and beauty vlogger Cassandra Bankson, who has suffered from acne for years and has perfected the art of covering it!)

Lastly, try to set your skepticism aside. You may think that essential oils are for the woo-woo, Neo-hippie crunchy type. But remember that before medicine as we know it today came to exist, everything was "natural". Plants had always been used (successfully) for their healing properties, and the fact that today they are labeled as "alternative" because we reach out for synthetic medicine that may work faster doesn't take away those properties.

So just approach your acne with an open mind and make sure that, no matter what you decide to heal it, you make an informed decision!

Chapter Two

The basic formula and how to use it.

Do you know about René-Maurice Gattefossé? His name may not seem familiar to you, but you've certainly heard the term he coined: aromatherapy. A French engineer and chemist coming from a family of perfumers (and so having grown up around producers of essential oils in the South of France), Gattefossé became severely burnt during an explosion in his laboratory. His wounds, treated with the conventional medicine of the time (it was in 1910, after all!), soon became gangrenous. As a last resort, he took off his bandages and intuitively poured lavender essential oil on his burns. The results were miraculous, and showed him that lavender oil had amazing antiseptic and cicatrising properties. It lead him to spend the rest of his life researching the healing properties of essential oils of plants and flowers.

Just like Gattefossé, I have found the effects of lavender oil to be nothing less than miraculous, healing my skin fast and more effectively than anything else I'd tried.

The main reason why I recommend the use of lavender essential oil in this book is because of its versatility. It kills acne-causing bacteria, reduces inflammation and dryness, and heals the skin, preventing severe scarring. On top of this, is also one of the most affordable essential oils; if you can only afford one oil, get lavender.

I use lavender oil for more than just skincare. I apply it to treat scraps, cuts and burns (which happen quite a lot because I'm a major klutz who loves nonetheless to cook and bake). I wear a few drops in my diffuser necklace, because it makes me feel calm and relax. I apply it on my hair to make it smell good. I also reach for my bottle of lavender essential oil whenever I get scratched by my cat (she only does it playfully!); it reduces the pain, heals the scratch in no time, and reduces any risk of infection.

My acne-healing formula comes in two parts: a topical treatment and a balm. In this chapter, I will give you the most basic formula to heal your acne. The fact that it is simple doesn't make it less potent or effective, but you have the option of using more ingredients, which I'll cover in the next chapter.

For now, all you need are two ingredients: lavender essential oil and coconut oil. I recommend getting the best you can afford from a reputable manufacturer: make sure the lavender oil is 100% pure and preferably organic. I trust Young Living and Aura Cacia for all my essential oils needs, but do your research before you decide who to buy from! As to coconut oil, I like it to be organic, virgin, cold-pressed and solid (the liquid form has gone through more processing). I find the one that meets all these requirements for $5.99 at Trader Joe's, but there are many more in most supermarkets, health food stores, and online.

For the topical treatment, simply use undiluted lavender oil. Pour a few drops of lavender oil into your clean hands, and apply it with your fingers to your pimples, blisters, and reddened areas. Or just apply it all over your face — I still do this twice a day even though my face is free from acne, as I find it evens out my complexion and keeps improving it. Follow the topical treatment by nourishing your skin with the coconut oil balm — we'll get to that in a bit.

This goes without saying, but only apply undiluted essential oil to your face if your skin can withstand it (which you can find out by testing it on a small area). If undiluted lavender oil causes your skin more harm than good, that's okay. Skip the topical treatment and move on straight to the balm.

The balm is your all-purpose moisturiser.
To make it, you'll need lavender oil, coconut oil, a clean and dry container with a lid, and a spoon to scoop it out without using your fingers which will have touched your face. I like to use a ratio of 50 drops of lavender oil for 1/2 cup of coconut oil, but you can use more or less depending on what you feel your skin needs.
Begin by melting the coconut oil, which is usually solid at room temperature. The best way to do it is by running the jar under hot water. Once it has become liquid, pour it out into your clean, dry container. Make sure it isn't boiling hot so the essential oil don't evaporate, then pour in the essential oil. Stir with your spoon and let the mixture solidify into a balm.

Apply this balm to your face morning and evening, and even during the day if it feels dry. Scoop out a pea-sized amount (a little goes a long way), melt it between your hands and apply it all over your face, especially wherever it feels particularly dry and irritated.

You can still use this balm under make-up. Just apply a smaller amount (add more if needed) and wait a few minutes for your skin to absorb it, then lightly and gently pat your face with a clean tissue and apply your makeup as usual.

This balm can be used to remove make-up as well, but if your eyes are sensitive, just use coconut oil on its own. Scoop out a quarter-sized amount and slather it on your face, drawing circles with the tips of your fingers to break down your makeup. Wipe it off with a tissue or a towel (you don't need any water, but you can run it under warm water if you like). Repeat multiple times, until the last wipe you use is completely clean.

Chapter Three

More ingredients.

The basic formula of lavender essential oil and coconut oil that we spoke about in the previous chapter works perfectly without the need to add any more ingredients. However, I'll be discussing in this chapter a few other essential oils and carrier oils that you can use if you want the option to try more ingredients and customise your formula. If you can afford these extra ingredients, by all means, get them and have fun with them! As long as you're not allergic or insensitive, natural ingredients can only bring more goodness to you. And, last but not least, essential oils smell delicious and will do wonders to your mood and mind!

Essential oils

Aside from lavender oil, there are other oils that I sometimes blend together and apply to my skin, either undiluted or mixed into a carrier oil. Here are the main five oils I like to have on hand to treat my skin:

Tea tree oil: You've more than likely heard about it in the past few years, since there has been countless lines of products made with tea tree oil and boasting its benefits. Tea tree oil has amazing antibacterial properties and works fast to dry out stubborn pimples. I recommend using it in its pure, undiluted form, so you don't have to put any artificial ingredients on your skin. Tea tree oil can be very astringent and harsh on some skin types, so I recommend applying a very small amount with a Q-tip on a pimple or blister.

Clary sage: I love clary sage because not only it helped reduce the appearance of my acne scars (I still see them, but only if I obsessively look in a magnifying mirror!), but it also reduces the excess production of sebum and prevents hormonal acne flare-ups from being severe. Lastly, it helps me cope with PMS symptoms, which is always a good thing.

Grapefruit essential oil: Remember the Neutrogena grapefruit scrub of your high school years? I'll admit what I like most about grapefruit oil is its delicious, citrusy scent (grapefruit is one of my favourite fruits, after all). Aside from lifting up your mood (which is important when you're coping with something as heavy as cystic acne!), grapefruit essential oil has antibacterial and antiseptic properties, and I always feel like my skin gets brighter when I use grapefruit oil! A word of caution: always ask your doctor if you're on any medication, since grapefruit can interfere with it.

Rosemary essential oil: Rosemary oil is often used for dry scalps, and whenever I apply it on my face, it gets less dry overnight. I also like that rosemary oil, whenever I use it, lifts up my mood and allows me to concentrate better

Frankincense essential oil: Frankincense, apart its wonderful spiritual uses, is great for skincare. It is antiseptic, as well as anti-inflammatory, and can help reduce wrinkles as well as fight acne (if you're an adult, you might as well start working on signs of age!).

A word about rose essential oil: do not buy cheap rose oil, since it's usually rose absolute, and not rose essential oil. Rose oil works really, really well, as much on the skin than on the mood, but is extremely expensive, so I'm not recommending it as a treatment oil here when more affordable oils work just as well. If you find natural products that contain rose essential oil, I more than recommend you use them!

Carrier oils

Sweet almond oil: When I was in high school, an Algerian friend's mom gave me a bottle of sweet almond oil, and I used it on my skin and hair. It smelled delicious and made my hair much softer and more luscious. I recommend mixing a few drops with your coconut oil or using it on its own as a moisturiser or makeup remover.

Olive oil: Olive oil has been used for hundreds of years by women in the Mediterranean as a moisturiser for the skin and hair. The only reason why I don't use olive oil 100% of the time is because I worry it might make me smell like a salad! But the smell can be masked if you mix it with essential oils, which is what I often do when I don't have coconut oil on hand and need a moisturiser/makeup remover.

Argan oil: Argan oil hails from North Africa, where it is used not just for beauty, but as a cooking oil as well. Real argan oil has a strong, delicious smell. You might know it through the "Moroccan Oil" brand, but I recommend you buy pure argan oil that hasn't been mixed with additives and other substances. It is on the more expensive side, but the benefits (great skin and soft hair and cuticles) are worth it.

Shea butter: My shea butter moisturiser from L'Occitane did help a lot when my skin was dry and angry, but years later, I found out I could have bought a large container of pure, unrefined shea butter from an African grocery store (or a health food store) for $4 instead of the 1oz jar that I had paid $40 for! Shea butter is the skincare secret my African friends' mothers all gave me when I asked them, astonished, what they did to look more like my friends' sisters than their mothers. Let's all agree that African women have the best skin in the world, so if you want to take skincare advice from anyone, it's from them!

Chapter Four

To pop or not to pop? *(Ew, eew, but like seriously, eeeeeewwwwww!!!)*

Do you feel the urge to pop that major, bigly, yuuuuge pimple? Here's what to do:

1. Lock yourself in your bathroom.
2. Turn off the lights.
3. Light two candles.
4. Repeat in the mirror "You are not a licensed dermatologist" as many times as it takes for you to be unpossessed from the urge to pop your pimples (it's very, very hard!).

Alternatively, you can tell yourself that for every pimple you pop, Jesus kills a kitten, a puppy and a baby hedgehog.

The urge to pop pimples is more psychological than anything else. We just want them gone, obliterated, and we think that this is the best way to do it. Also, let's just admit that pimple-popping is disgustingly satisfying (everyone who ever popped a huge cyst can attest to that).

You've gathered that I'm not going to recommend popping pimples in this book, even if I confess having done it way more times than I should have. I have a few scars on my cheeks, forehead and chin, that are only visible on a magnifying mirror, but I know they're there nonetheless because I popped many of my huge puss-filled blisters, sometimes before they even came to a head. Popping acne puts a lot of pressure on the skin, especially if you try to dig out a pimple with your nails (that's the worst, and I've got the scars to prove it). Popping is also the best way for bacteria to get into the open sore and cause infection and more acne.

If you still decide to pop your pimples, here's what not to do:
Don't pop any pimple with your bare nails (wrap your fingers in clean tissue), without washing your hands or skin before.
Don't skip following up with the topical treatment (if you pop, make sure you apply one of the aforementioned essential oils to prevent bacteria from spreading and to reduce the inflammation and swelling!).
Don't use any towels, especially dirty ones. Only use clean tissues or gauze if you have any; the key is to be as hygienic as you would if you were performing surgery (since you're essentially cutting into your skin, making it vulnerable to infection).

Don't pop any pimples that haven't come to a head (that's the best way to make the pimple last longer and cause permanent damage to your skin).
Don't pop blackheads if they can't easily fall off with light exfoliation: it's better to get a facial or use a peel-off mask.

The best alternative to popping is to view the blemish as a part of your own skin (as opposed as a parasite that needs to be removed), reacting the way it does because it is under aggression. Instead of obliterating it, try nurturing it so it can heal. Apply lavender oil or your topical treatment blend regularly, until the blemish either swells down and fades, or dries out and falls off on its own. And then, make sure to nurture the raw, exposed skin underneath as much as possible.

Chapter Five

Lifestyle changes.

We've covered the basic formula that will heal your acne topically. It may be the main thing to do, but it is not the only one. I'd be lying if I told you that was all there is to it. The thing is, healing your acne has to come from the inside as well as what you put on your skin. A healthy diet, exercise, and reducing stress are all major factors in improving the quality of your skin. The good news is, these changes will not only help your acne, but improve your quality of life and lead you to feel healthier, have more energy, and feel better in your mind.

The importance of eating better:

Eliminate processed foods from your diet. This is one of the most important changes to make if you want your skin to heal. When I ate processed foods, I broke out much more than when I cut them out from my diet. While there hasn't been enough research yet to prove that food additives and preservatives cause breakouts (let alone ruin our health overall), it doesn't take a degree in biochemistry to see the correlation between processed foods and acne and other health issues. So be mindful as a consumer of what harmful ingredients are snuck into your food, and make an informed decision as to what you eat.

Eat lots fruits and vegetables. Try to buy organic produce if it is accessible and affordable to you (check Costco, discount food stores like Aldi, and farmers' markets - seasonal and local produce is always less expensive). I don't advocate going vegetarian or vegan (because it's your own personal decision to make), but try as much as you can to make fruits and vegetables your main dish. I like to have a large bowl of fruit for breakfast (the vitamins!) along with a little bit of bread, cheese and eggs. For lunch, I have either a large lettuce or arugula salad (seasoned with lemon juice and olive oil - salad dressing is so fatty and has not-so-good ingredients!) or a plate of steamed or roasted veggies with a small side of pasta, rice or meat. For dinner, I always have vegetable soup - I either buy the organic boxed soup from Trader Joe's (to which I add spices), or make my own veggie soup on Sunday, store it in the fridge, and reheat it throughout the week.

Eat less of the foods that cause you acne. To my biggest dismay, cheese makes me break out. I'm French, so I still eat it (it will take a lot more than acne to take away my love for cheese!), but in much smaller amounts nowadays and mostly around my period (if I'm going to break out anyways… #pragmatism). Also, I noticed that artisan cheese imported from France (or from small producers in this country) causes me less breakouts than processed cheese bought from the cheese aisle at the store; I believe it has to do with the quality of ingredients used and the absence of additives and preservatives. And let's not even talk about that orange plastic cheese product atrocity I refuse to call "American cheese" because I love America (it is my country as much as France!) and believe it can do much better than this in terms of cheese! Another thing I noticed triggers my acne is meat (perhaps it has to do with the hormones in it?). I love meat and ham, but I've been eating it very occasionally and in small amounts.

Drink lots of water. Water is life. Water flushes out toxins from our bodies, and helps our skin cells renew. Water hydrates your skin from the inside, and remember what we said about dryness being a cause of acne? The general recommendation is to drink eight cups of water a day, but I need more than that. I drink from my refillable 32-oz water bottle, which I fill about three to four times a day and carry everywhere with me. Some of us use apps to track your water intake; for me it isn't necessary since I don't need to force myself to drink water, but the tools to take your health in hand are out there for you to use should you need them!

Consume less sugar. Just like oil, sugar isn't evil in itself. But anything in excess can cause health problems, and sugar is snuck into processed foods, especially in America, causing our palates to become too used to the sweet taste (I personally cut the sugar amounts in half in all American recipes I try). Try to consume sugar mindfully, treating it as a pleasure rather than a given. For example, I would rather skip sugary drinks (see my next point) and enjoy a delicious slice of flourless dark chocolate cake instead.

Replace soft drinks with sparkling mineral water. Soft drinks contain artificial colourings and flavours, and unhealthy amounts of sugar. The diet versions aren't better (and believe me, I'm a recovering Diet Coke addict), because they're filled have not-so-good artificial sweeteners instead. Sparkling water is a healthier alternative, and it can help you wean yourself off the sugary taste (see previous point). Mineral water contains ingredients that are amazing for the skin, and the bubbles feel festive, a bit like Champagne!

Talking of Champagne, drink alcohol in moderation. There's no need to cut off alcohol, but enjoy it as an occasional treat and don't binge (in other words, don't get drunk and use it as an excuse to pop your pimples!). Alcohol dilates the blood vessels in your skin, making it more red. There are claims that some ingredients in certain types of alcoholic drinks can make acne worse. As I said previously, consume with moderation and listen to your body and how it reacts to what you feed it.

Drink tea! Try to reduce your coffee intake, as it tends to dehydrate the skin. I'm not saying cut off caffeine entirely (God forbid!), but try to have one or two cups of espresso or americano in the morning and as an afternoon pick-me-up, and drink tea throughout the day instead. Black, green and white tea all have excellent health benefits. But Rooibos, an herbal tea made from a south-African red bush (hence the name), is by definition the perfect tea to heal acne and improve your skin's appearance. It doesn't contain caffeine, so it can be drunk at any time throughout the day and in large amounts.

Enjoy quality foods that make you happy, in moderation. This is the key to eating well for your skin and health. Avoid excesses and buy the best quality foods you can afford. It will help heal your acne and have wonderful effects on your health and life.

Exercise:

Exercise flushes out the toxins from your body, helps you maintain a healthy weight and keep your muscles and joints in good shape. It also raises your endorphins, making you happier (and better mood = good!).

I've never been a big fan of exercise (to answer your question as to why this paragraph is shorter than the other two in this chapter), until I found out forms of it that make me happy. Do what makes you happy. I love to **walk** (to meet the needs of a high-energy dog and to keep my bragging rights for high Fitbit numbers!), **swim** in the ocean when the weather allows it (saltwater and iodine are miraculous with acne!), and do several hours of **yoga** per week. I won't go into the benefits of yoga here because they'll probably make this book five times longer, but yes, out of the many wonderful effects yoga had on my life, improving my skin was one of them, so I definitely recommend you try it! If yoga isn't for you, just find *your thing*: you can run, dance, surf, anything to raise those endorphins levels!

Eliminating stress:

Bathe or shower to relax. Water is so therapeutic and easily accessible. I love taking a nice bubble bath at the end of a long day, with lots of lavender oils and bath salts and, pleasure of all pleasures, a scented bath bomb from Lush. While it may not be the eco-friendliest thing, I do many other things to help the environment and indulge into this bathing ritual that sucks away the stress from my body and mind. If you don't have a bathtub, don't despair: you can transform your shower into a perfect stress-relieving oasis by following the steps listed on my blog, **agirlwitharedbag.wordpress.com.**

Try yoga and meditation. No, this isn't a book about the benefits of yoga (but stay tuned because that book is coming), but yoga and meditation have this magical way of melting the stress away and filling your body and soul with love and self-worth.

Get reiki or lay on a Biomat. Reiki, or energy healing, can not only reduce stress, but it helps to cure physical ailments as well. Try to find a practitioner near you and give it a try; you won't regret it. The Biomat, a gemstone-filled infrared mat that you lie down on, is a worthy investment because it literally sucks out the stress from your body and fills you with peace and relaxation. You can find a Reiki practitioner near you who owns one you can try.

Remove sources of stress. When I quit a job that was making me unhappy and barely paying enough for me to make ends meet (after I'd found a better job!), my skin improved drastically. When I distanced myself from negative people, cutting off the worst of them (with that good old "unfriend" button), my skin healed even faster. People can be so negative and we don't always notice how much they can bring us down. While there are ways to tune out the negativity of people you are forced to see on a daily basis, the best is to just peacefully walk away.

See a therapist if you can afford it. Consider talking to one online, as it is usually less expensive. While you suffer from severe acne, you are vulnerable and need the professional support of someone who will listen to you, give you sound advice, and put things in perspective for you. Don't let yourself sink into depression because of the stigma around acne.

Don't isolate yourself. Cover your acne with makeup and create a smokey eye or a bold red lip. Put your best clothes on and get out of the house. Spend time with close friends you love and trust, people who will know better than to make you feel self-conscious about your skin, but rather be tactful and only offer support or advice when solicited.

Tune out the nasty comments. I still remember that one time at a friend's birthday party, when a girl insisted to do my portrait and then, when she was done drawing me, said, "now I can add a pimple here, and one here, and another here." She probably thought she was being funny, but I got upset. Another time, an older coworker publicly humiliated me (but mostly herself), touching my face, rubbing off my makeup with her fingers, then saying (very loud) that I wouldn't have any acne if I just washed my face. And I'll never forget that memorable occasion where, at a large family gathering, a near-stranger took me aside and asked me whether I had a boyfriend, adding that having lots of sex would cure my acne. After all these incidents, I wondered if someone would ever offer to sacrifice a chicken under the full moon for my skin to improve. The point is, some people won't know how to butt out and mind their own business. So the only thing you can do is not take their comments personally but rather smile, thank them for their advice, and change the subject or walk away.

Know that your skin will heal. It's only a matter of time. Skin regenerates itself, and acne is skin that needs to be treated differently from the inside out. Acne isn't cancer, diabetes, HIV, or any other incurable, chronic condition. It can and will be healed by the changes you make in your skincare regimen and overall lifestyle. You will run across fatalistic posts online from people who feel desperate (which is normal and legitimate). I used to read those posts from people who tried so many different cures and still didn't heal their acne, and I would feel even more depressed and hopeless. I was proven wrong thanks to my nearly-miraculous healing formula, and I hope for your own sake you'll spare yourself what I put myself through and instead sleep with the knowledge that your skin will heal, and it isn't a question of *if* but rather *when*.

Conclusion

Dear reader,

Thank you for reading my book; I hope you found it informative and useful. Please don't hesitate to share your feedback by reviewing it, and reach out to me if there's something you'd like to add!

In this book, I tried to cover the topic of acne as broadly as possible with the goal of keeping this a quick and coherent read. I encourage you to research any topics more extensively if you are seeking precise information on them.

As I write those final words, I hope that you will give my method a try and that it will work as wonderfully for you as it did for me. I hope that your acne will once be nothing more than a distant memory and a story you can tell in turn to help others.

I will repeat it as many times as necessary - make an informed decision before following any course of treatment, be it conventional or alternative. We're privileged to live in the internet era, so don't hesitate to put this wonderful tool to use!

And please, try not to dismiss natural treatments as "alternative" or "woowoo". While there may be snake oil scammers out there, all they do is dissuade people from natural healing by discrediting it. Try to use your own judgment: nature is one big, bountiful and efficient pharmacy - let's not turn our backs to it now that we have modern medicine. Scientific progress and ancient therapies should work hand-in-hand rather than be at war against one another.

I hope this method will work for you, and I hope you don't get discouraged if it doesn't. Something **will** work. You can overcome this, so don't lose hope: acne is only temporary

Lastly, know that you are beautiful. Even with your acne, you are beautiful, and this is an irrefutable truth. I hope this can raise your self-esteem and give you hope.

Love,

Marie.

PS: for more information and a list of resources, visit **agirlwitharedbag.wordpress.com** and follow me on Instagram @agirlwitharedbag.